The Unlimited Self

Get to know yourself, feel free and satisfied in one month!!!

You've probably read a lot of smart books on how to become happy, how to improve ourselves ...

What I suggest is not a panacea, but it is tested, verified and gives results. Our society is so developed that requires from us daily efforts, learning and adjustment . Somewhere in our everyday life happiness-such as we imagined it when we were teens - disappears . The road to happiness passes through the knowledge of ourselves, our body, emotions and life.

The physical body is the temple of our soul. Everyone knows the phrase "Healthy body, healthy mind"! That is why to be completed, it is important to care, appreciate and know our own body. We have to do the best we are capable of and to recognize and respect any sign that it gives us, something we can do about it.

When you feel comfortable in your body you feel strength, energy and confidence leading to a life, full of joy, harmony and satisfaction.

You enjoy your own well-being, which enables you to be a loving and equal partner in any relationship; you feel confidence and fulfillment. You have complete freedom to be yourself, without any dependence on the opinions and approval of others. Circumstances do not become a creator and performer of our own destiny.

Each of us knows how we loose energy and desire for life when we do not feel comfortable in our body. "Wow, I grow fat! "or" Wow, my nose is ugly!" We have a feeling of failure, of imperfection. We believe that we are not worthy to be loved and enjoyed. We do not have the necessary power and resources to achieve what we want and we do not know what will make us truly happy. The truth is that we can learn to use and accept what the Universe has given us - such opportunities and resources to find and achieve the easiest way to balance the happiness in every moment of our life situation. That   means that we can change it,

improve it, and   accept it for now and with this confidence to strive for new goals and successes. Doesn`t all this sound like a desire or a difficult task ?! Patience, as it says in the Bible, is one of the human virtues!

Astrology is one of the most ancient sciences that gives us answers to all vital questions we face daily in our lives. It helps us to find the most direct route to the objective that we have set in this incarnation. Not surprisingly, in ancient times, kings, rulers, philosophers and psychologists have even trusted the strength and power of the planets and their impact on us. They observed them and complied with their terms and combinations, used their guidance, favourable influences and received moments in which their unfavourable combination gave them signs to have patience, acceptance and humility before a higher power with absolute confidence in it and in its infinite precision and justice!

Not in vain, participants in the elections for local government all over the world visit astrologers to find out whether they will be successful in the struggle for power.

Each zodiac sign gives a unique ability and knowledge to the individual - to use our strength, to know our weaknesses. It indicates which parts of the body are vulnerable in this life and if we watch them and be reckoned with small limitations that each of us has, we can go through life with ease and gratitude to fate and the Universe.

Astrology is the place where past, present and future meet!

One of the inalienable facts ,that we have provided, is consciousness and free will to make reasonable choices and take full responsibility for them in every unique moment and situation happening in our present life.

There is no right and wrong, not correct and incorrect. The truth is that conscience is the best and

perfect criterion for everything that we go through and experience fully consciously in our life.

The purpose of this reading is to give us a boost on the way to our personal happiness and if reading the last lines we feel peace, harmony and a sense of lightness deep inside, the choice we have made is the right and proper for us at this moment. For each of us this choice may be different, but it only can   show us that the world is colourful and varied; people are unique individuals who, according to their family environment and education, society and moral foundations in which grow, build and follow a system of values and a different approach to perception and experience of the world.

This does not make any of us better or worse, more successful or unsuccessful, happier or more miserable! It shows that diversity should be respected and accepted with tolerance and understanding and, above all, empathy. The only thing that unites all people in the world, regardless of race, religion and society, is the internal feeling of lightness that comes from a clear conscience.

Happy people have a gleam in the eye. You want to have some of their tranquility and confidence. "All happy people are alike" – That is true! The purpose of the book is to help you go one step towards your success as individuals, as parents, as employees or bosses, to help you accept yourself and   find new ways to prosperity!

The exercises I have suggested will give you freedom and independence to be "just yourselves," wherever you are on your way. They reveal your ability to create, to leave trails after your existence, to be an example for your children and their children; to give the world the best of which we are capable, without any conditions, because this is our inner desire that makes us happy and satisfied.

Later in the book you will find and be able to use theoretical and practical exercises, tips and hints on how to balance and fill your physical and spiritual body with strength, positive energy, creativity and a sense of wholeness. This does not mean you'll never have problems, trials or you will not feel pain. This is not the purpose of this book. We are here to learn, develope and improve, and always go through trials. What is written here can help you and teach you how to go through these events without leaving you physically and emotionally exhausted for a long period of time. When we are deeply hurt we usually blame someone else or something for what happens to us!

This book will enable you to understand and accept everything as a blessing and as an uncut diamond. If we consider any situation or event, and analyze it and look impartially with the eyes of an outsider, we can express our most sincere thanks to the Universe for its unique and fair nature, that everything is accurate and most perfectly for each of us.

Lastly, one of the most important conditions for internal and external balance, is the maintenance and care of our physical body. It is the main thing from which we start our journey. When it is combined with inner awareness, which can be achieved through certain meditative practices and exercises for just several minutes a day, you will achieve absolute wonders for a very short period of time.

PART 1

MAGIC MOON

The moon is "light" we need when it is"dark"! It shows our subconscious intention. Though it is a scientific absurd, researchers revealed a deep psychological truth   -   that in our busy lives (logical and rational), oriented almost to the sun, we do not really
manage to maintain the harmony. Simbolically, the moon represents less conscious side of human existence and sometimes we see just in its diffused light more clearly than in the glare of the sun (sun sign)!

The Moon is called the "soul of life." Without it, we would have only the mechanical and tireless performance, which in the end of all is without cultural interests! Without moon we would have no poetry, literature, art, music, dance and dreams.

Artists are famous for their "dreaminess" and we all also dream   when the night reigns over us.

Moon phases affect each of us with great power and strength. If we can use this power we can create a lot more happiness in life than we can imagine!

We will use one of the phases of the moon - "new moon". Phase which allows us to set up every our desire and purpose. So, follow these steps from the beginning of the "new moon".

Here you can see the "new moons" of 2016:

January 9 Capricorn 20; 31;

February 8 Aquarius 9:40;

March 8 Pisces 20: 56;

April 7 Aries 06: 24 ;

May 6 Taurus 14: 30 ;

June 4 Gemini 22: 01;

July 4 Cancer 06: 02;

August 2 **Leo** 15: 45;

September 1 Virgin 04: 04;

September 30 Libra 19: 13;

October 30 Skorpion 12: 39 ;

November 29 Sagittarius   07: 19 ;

December 29 Capricorn   01: 55 ;

What I suggest is a month-long program that can improve your life and make it more interesting, more satisfied. The new self-assessment will help you to give yourself and your relatives and friends around you love and happiness.

Start the program when it is a "new moon". The influence of the moon is the most strongly during the first eight hours, so define and record your goals during these hours.

Define one goal or desire on every "new moon", thus you will concentrate the energy in one aim. You can also

start with the first step and try to formulate a purpose a few days before the "
new moon". The aim must be quite clear for you when you put it down in the log in the time of "new moon".

1st step: we look at ourselves and evaluate the condition in which we find ourselves at this very moment - feelings, thoughts, emotions, desires

2nd step: Determining and setting a target that we would follow if we decide to change something.

3rd step: Create a mantra that symbolizes our goal.

4th step: Consciously determine the resources that we have and the time we will spend to achieve our goal.

5th step: The most difficult - To accept ourselves as we are at   present

6th step: Creating a healthy diet that accompanies the objective.

7th step: Studying and application of meditative practices and exercises.

8th step: Reporting the results and achievements of the work and our efforts

9th **step** - the most important – we appreciate and reward ourselves for the success.

The following pages will address each step in order to be of help to anyone who has decided to take a unique journey to its profound essence in building a happier person.

FIRST STEP

Alone, without any help, make self-assessment that gives you a clear idea of the state you are at present. This step is very important in order to give a clear idea of what is "here and now" and it will allow us to set clear goals in the next steps to follow.

For example, yesterday a client was deeply surprised by her self- assessment. She said that she has always thought of herself as a good, responsive and pitiful person, but sitting down with a pen and paper in hand to write she actually found that the words "good" and "compassionate" somehow do not want to appear on the leaves. She was irritated by the discovery and was about to lose self-confidence.

So my dear men and women, do not need to judge and condemn if you are not perfect or sinless. It is important to approach realistic and be aware to what it is now, right now, in this situation. Remember, that you are not the only ones who are worried or have something you like or dislike. It happens to everyone whether you see it in others or not. Give yourself all the time and space for this to be yourself, just yourself. As you are right now.!

EXERCISE 1

Buy a small notebook and name it whatever you want, "John", "Tina" ... put it on a convenient place for you. Then sit or lie down where you feel relaxed and comfortable and feel your whole body. Do not hurry, do not force the things. Follow your inner impulse. Give yourself the time you need to adjust and relax without worrying. Close your eyes for a moment and turn your attention inward of you. Take a few deep breaths and with each exhalation feel relax and remain still. Give yourself all the love that you are capable of at this time and allow it to hug you entirely.

Focus in the so called "third eye" - it is on your forehead between the eyes. Stay as an impartial observer of everything that comes or goes there. These can be pictures, memories or feelings, lights. Do not analyze, just watch. Some of them bring you the feeling of pain, discomfort, sadness. Do not run away from them. Let them and allow them to be part of you. Follow the pictures and sensations.

Let your movie go ahead. Be a spectator. Feel moments that give and receive love, those in which you allow yourself to be innocent, you might see yourself as a child or grown-up - just observe and follow them!

Give yourself all the time you need and wait while the paintings begin to fade. Then take again a few deep breaths and carefully (when you are ready to start) move your body. First shake your fingers and toes, then simply stretch.

Take your journal and write down everything you think important and valuable to save in it. That will allow you to express aloud these situations and feelings that you do not want to admit and which sometimes scare you.

It'll show you those experiences that bring you joy and love without even doubt. It seems easy, right?

Do this exercise every 5-6 days for 30 days. The exercise can be done alone or in combination with the following ones.

Only in this way you will relieve and take in your heart your true nature, as it is without judgment or blame. Everything we try to escape comes again with bigger strength, just as we have decided that we have forgotten or thrown away from us. All we can do is to allow those feelings and emotions be part of us .
Thus we agree with the fate and allow it to take care for us in
the best way. We can afford us to be weak and vulnerable sometimes, we will be willing to trust ourselves and the loved ones, which is the most direct route to feel love and closeness. Nevertheless, we are sometimes hurt we can move forward with new confidence and fate!!!

2ND STEP

Determining and setting a target that we would follow if we decide to change something.

This step is important to determine what currently makes us feel uncomfortable. This could be our body, our relationships, our sense of uncertainty, our career, income, loss of a loved one or something else.

Select this one thing on which to work in the next one month If there is more than one thing you want to change focus only on what your thoughts go back whenever you're at rest. Leave the other factors for your
discomfort for the coming months. Remember that writing of the purpose must be in the first eight hours of the "new moon".

The subconscious of human beings acts intuitively and it has no ability to analyze. It is important to give it a clear objective on which to adjust, focus and work. You must be aware that the subconscious mind of man is a powerful tool for change. Everything coded in it properly leads to materialization of life. Some years ago, I was one of those people who do not believe that the thought of man can define and determine what is happening. But my experience has proven over time that I have been on "the dark side of the moon" - misguided.

Choose consciously each goal. Remember that it is important to believe, think and feel positive and be persistent in this direction. It can start with a small and an easier target at the beginning. This will give you the confidence and courage that you can deal with larger goals.

In the following rows I will give examples how to determine and follow targets:

If you need confidence can set the following purpose:

"I accept and love myself unconditionally"

If you want to fight with any habit you can put the following purpose.

"I want my desire to smoke to leave me in the coming days."

If you want to improve your professional realization you can paste the following purpose:

"I want the next month to find and follow every idea that will help me to grow in the professional field."

If you need to improve your relationship:

"I want to find the most correct approach to my partner, which leads to harmony in our relationship."

If you want to improve your health you may write:

"I want my body to be absolutely healthy and full of energy."

Let's start!

EXERCISE 1

You can start doing this exercise a few days or a week before the "new moon". Even if there is no very clear purpose that day, do not worry. Maybe the aim requires a little more time to clarify or the moment may need a little more time. **Remember** that everything happens at the "right place at the right time"!

Take your journal and sit comfortably. Close your eyes and relax. Take a few deep breaths and exhale calmly and gently. Give yourself the time needed to relax and clear your mind. When you feel peace and harmony in yourself start to ask yourself the following question for at least 5 minutes: "What I need at this moment to feel happy?"

Do not analyze and do not think if what comes to your mind is right or wrong. Let your thoughts come and go. Try to feel the answer that is the most appropriate for you at this time. It is very likely that you get a message that you have thought about.

But our feeling is the exact source of what we need at any moment. So trust your inner feeling and and let me guide you and develop your most perfect and hidden potential.

When you come across this objective clearly and precisely in mind, check how you feel in your body. If your aim is right, the body will feel relaxed, calm and without any tension. Do the exercise not less than 20

minutes. After the end of it put in the diary everything that emerged spontaneously: images, words, situations, colours, smell...

Some of you may need more time to reach a clear objective, but this must t not bother you. Everything happens for everyone at the right time. So do the exercise as much as it needed. Be sure that at the moment when you clearly formulate and define your purpose, is the moment in which you assume and open new paths to prosperity and happiness.

Make the exercise as many days as needed until you feel within yourself that the objective is the most appropriate in the current situation. When you find it get the diary and record on a new page in large letters clear, concise and accurate on which you will focus the next one month.

For example:
"I want to attract happiness and harmony in my life "
"I want to find the right job for me."
"I want a new relationship with the most appropriate partner"
"I want to improve my financial situation"
"I want perfect health"

A lot of women want everything now and immediately. Do not be too ambitious! Who needs this?! Listen to yourself, in the so called sixth sense, to your inner voice and choose what is the most important to you now at the present moment.

3RD STEP

Creating a mantra, which symbolizes our goal.
Creating mantra is essential for the success because
our subconscious mind is naturally pure and selfless
and

it needs a code to restructure essence, to reach and
to get materialized in our lives.

It is important to find the shortest positive form which
defines our purpose. You may find it difficult to get
just one answer. If more, do not them simultaneously
but consequently . In the following lines I will give
examples how to create your mantra.

If you want happiness you can decrypt "I am happy "
If you want to increase your income: "I grow rich"
If you want good health: "I am healthy"

The mantra that you create for this purpose
must be positive and in the present tense. It is

encoded in the subconscious and it accepts it as already occurring. Therefore it is necessary to be short and clear. Repeat it as many times as you remember a day for the entire period in which you work on the purpose.

Do not change or replace it until it becomes part of you. Close your eyes and say: I am healthy!

4TH STEP

Consciously determining the resource that we have and the time we will spend to achieve our goal.

This step is the step that will make the goal real - the goal that you have already discovered and felt in yourself. It is important to define the time you want and you can take, to follow the goal you set.

From my personal experience I know that if you start with a small goal it is easier. It is not necessary to have huge goals in the beginning. This can discourage you, but this is not our goal, right? Performance of practices and exercises should give us pleasure and do not get tired. So, determine how much time will you will spend and try to follow it. You can do it as a game with your children or loved ones that will bring not only satisfaction, but also a joyful experience.

My advice is to start with a simple purpose to feel the force and energy that goes off whenever you want. But if you set a large goal, or one that has no time to delay, it requires greater competence. Well, to find the appropriate consultant. For example, if your goal is to cure a disease it is necessary in any case to consult the appropriate professional or do the necessary research. The program must be professionally made.

Always combine mental, physical and emotional in you. We are a full unity. So that only the combination will bring real results. Sometimes this balance is difficult, but if you have strong will the miracle, for which you have not even suspected, can happen. I know it's not as easy as it is to hear or read about it, but the truth is that it is not so impossible. At the moment you feel it and accomplish it you will be surprised by yourself . The first time is always the hardest.

5TH STEP

To accept ourselves as we are at present

The point of this step is to know and agree that there is no other time than "here and now" and that everything is happening at present. We must not miss the true gifts that life reveals to us with unconditional love. There may be things that worry us and we are not satisfied by them, but the truth is that they are all past experiences or future assumptions. It is very important to realize that!

We are unable to change neither past nor future at this moment, but we can agree with them.We must experience the present moment with full awareness and take responsibility for everything that happens to us. Try to look with loving heart and trust at yourself and at life. Even if we made some mistakes we should forgive ourselves and admit that we are an ordinary human being who is entitled to mistakes.

Actually, this is the only way to develop and improve ourselves. Only someone who makes mistakes can get wiser, learning from his/her own mistakes. Everyone should know that the real will and free choice of the people is expressed only when they have the courage to risk and take steps. regardless of the fear that it overwhelms them.

Fear is a normal human state of mind and without it we could not survive. It is important to move beyond this fear and allow ourselves   be vulnerable, fragile and with an open heart. Only in this way we will feel alive. Love, harmony, and happiness will come with them!

Fate and confidence in our own strength, value and capacity is the most powerful tool to achieve a good self-esteem, which will help us to feel confident! It will allow us to pursue our goals, dreams and longings with the flair of a researcher!

Practical guidelines and exercises related to the fifth step.

Exercise 1

You can record everything that happens to you in that month, day and night in your diary - every success, everything you discover about yourself, everything new and   old, everything you want to keep or want to change.

Do this exercise 30 days. Every morning or evening sit for 5-10 minutes in a quiet environment and start counting 15-20 positive qualities that you possess. Remember - only positive!   This exercise is for positive qualities. We will consider the others later!

You may repeat some of them (it does not matter), others will emerge with time, some of them will change. So, do not analyze! Do not use only your mind! Just write all that emerges. They can be related with your character, your professional realization or relationships. Write down all of them when they come to mind or when you feel them.

For example: I'm a good company, ... I have a sense of humor, I'm caring, I am loving and gentle, I'm nice, I'm spontaneous, I'm good at my job, I am a good daughter, etc....

Write down everything that comes as a thought in your mind and when you are in everyday life remember and repeat some of them as often as possible. This will bring you satisfaction and fill you with energy during the day.

Exercise 2

Find a quiet and calm space in your home which you can use the next 20 minutes. Stand up slowly and smoothly feel your body, feel your legs, arms, head or any part of it. Let your inner voice to guide you. Slowly start moving in free space without considering or analysing your movements. Let your inner intuition to guide you and just follow it.

What do you need to feel comfortable? You may need to stop, turn around, raise your hand, laugh. Just feel free and follow the impulse that comes in you without using your mind. Do not rush, explore anything that haunts you at this time. Enjoy the spontaneity over the next few minutes. Detect the time. Let your intuition to guide you and just naturally follow it.

When you feel that your body needs relax, find a suitable place that is convenient for you and just sit or lie down. Close your eyes and turn your attention to your heart chakra and observe. Take a few deep breaths and visualize in the heart area how the lotus blooms, which endows you with love and brightness. You can imagine that huge ball of white light fills you.

Visualize or if it is difficult to see it, you can just express it with words in a voice. It does not matter how you do it. It is important to feel how your whole body is filled with this light and you are part of it. Let it bring you enjoyment and peace, to fill you with a white glow and to purify you.

Merge with it and give yourself the space you need now. Stay as long as you need to feel it. When you are ready, gently and softly begin to return. Do not hurry! Enjoy the quiet and gentle serenity and privacy. Thank yourself. When you are ready you can move your body and open your eyes.

Do this exercise for 30 consecutive days. If you interrupt it you must start over to countdown. It is important to begin feeling your own body all the time and you allow it to lead you and guide you. This is a very good way to find and follow your own desires, aspirations and attitudes. It will help you feel comfortable, in harmony with yourself. It gives you the confidence and belief that what you want at any given moment is what you want internally, without hesitation or even doubt...

You will feel calm and balanced. This exercise can be done alone or in combination with the previous one. If you need or feel well you can practice it a few times a day. The exercise is very suitable when we feel vulnerable and stressed in our everyday life. It helps when we are in a state of discomfort or we are scared. You can use it when you're with other people. In these cases simply remain seated and just revel your body,

shake it and find the posture and position that will give you a sense of calm and confidence. . .

6TH STEP

Creating a healthy diet that accompanies the objective

It is very important to take care of the physical body which is the "temple of the soul". Love and acceptance are the main things that make us calm and help us feel confident. Even if you want to change something, the first thing you should do is to say "yes" to the current situation.

This is important because in this way you will not waste your energy on everyday concerns and convictions - energy that can be used to achieve everything imaginable in mind.Healthy eating and exercises provide energy, health and sense of confidence.

We believe that everything we do in our daily life is more or less a habit that we have created and which has become a part of our nature(in most of the cases unconsciously). A lot of our habits come from the environment in which we lived or from our parents. The good news is that each of these habits can be replaced by other that will meet our conscious choice.

The next 30 days try to be an experimenter of yourself. Find physical activities that bring you inner satisfaction and make them three times a week. If you do not have enough time to visit a gym or group classes you can make exercises yourself at home for 40 minutes at least 3 times a week.

I recommend you Yoga or Pilates which are relevant activities. They help both our physical body and internal balance for relaxation. Try to be consistent with the exercises.
The other essential thing is to follow a diet.

I will list some basic rules for nutrition:

1. Eat regularly - 3-4 times a day (hours)
2. Avoid heavy and fatty foods (examples)
3. Try to eat less meat during these 30 days.

4. Change meat with fish or fishery products if possible.

5. Let fruits and vegetables are your main menu. Freshly squeezed fruit juices are incredible for your metabolism. Make juice of your favorite fruits.

6. Avoid fried fast food - This is the most difficult part. It is difficult to me, too. I love fries and burgers, but they make me happy just for a moment. When I do not eat them and eat salads and soups instead ... satisfaction from the food by itself is multiplied many times!

7. Eat slowly and with love - it is also difficult, too!

And how to achieve it, especially at noon, when we have 30 or 40 minutes to eat and then we hurry to return to work ?! Eat with people who are pleasant to you!

8. Do not eat if you are furious and angry. Food becomes toxic when taken under the influence of

negative emotions. Do not eat when your heart is sad and stressed.

Drink a cup of almost hot water with some lemon - composure will follow.

9. Try to eat slowly and with relish, without being in a hurry. Perhaps, you've heard that every bite should be chewed at least 20 times. This is needed in order not to impede the work of the stomach.

10. Consume plenty of water (at least 2 liters a day and more if you like it) - it can purify your body and mind.

11. Avoid alcohol consumption. Well, I am so mean, aren`t I? I do not say that it is forbidden. Just limit it. You can sometimes drink a glass of wine or beer. Take care of yourself as of a loved one. Give the best to your body and know that it will thank you with a perfect health.

Exercise 1

The practice requires 3-4 minutes a day (in the morning and in the evening)

In the morning, before leaving for work, stay at rest (sitting or standing) for 3-4 minutes. Close your eyes and imagine that you are surrounded by a ball of light. It is hugging you and you feel its warmth and protection. State your desire to be surrounded by it throughout the day. When you are ready, open your eyes and stay with this energy all day long.

In the evening (before you go to bed) close your eyes again for 3-4 minutes and imagine that you are in front of a warm fresh waterfall. Feel the air, take a deep breath and exhale. Visualize how gently you enter the water and it washes all unnecessary things from you. When you feel purified, leave the vision to fade slowly. Then you can comfortably relax and get asleep.

7TH STEP

Studying and application of meditative practices and exercises

This step will help to balance your entirety. You can achieve miracles when you combine it with exercises and a diet.

Meditative practices are necessary so that everyone can feel the true nature without conditionalities, which we carry within ourselves. I will offer you a meditation practice which you can use every day for 30 days. If you decide then proceed with it further.

The practice is short, but very powerful. Make it the morning after awakening or at bedtime for 5-7 minutes. If you want you can make it in the morning and in the evening.

<u>Meditation practice</u>:

Relax in the supine position with palms up, feet shoulder-width apart. Close your eyes and take several deep breaths. Relax your body as much as possible.

Repeat 3 times out loud or mentally the mantra that you created in the previous step. Try to feel it in your body. When you are ready, imagine that you are where your goal is a reality. Feel the power and happiness that fills you from the achieved goal.

If you want a new job visualize your workplace, your colleagues who friendly smile to you friendly; feel the satisfying feeling that fills you because of the approval of others for your undeniable qualities, your successes and achievements!

If you want to improve your relationship with your partner you can visualize a nice place, which is a favourite one for both of you. See how gently you are touching your hands,feel the love that is there between you. Allow yourself to feel it and accept it. Feel how you two merge into one, full of harmony, balance, acceptance and love.

If you fail to visualize do not worry! You may need a little more practice.

It is important to feel the power and the limitless abilities which you carry and hold in your body. When you are ready to say aloud "I am a winner" take a deep breath, open your eyes and stay all day with the thought and the feeling that you are a winner.

Another practice that I use is to write the goal you have set on small notes and take them everywhere with you. You can

stick them at home or at work, to see them throughout the day. This allows you to stay in constant contact with
your goal. These simple practices are very strong and if you practice them long time you will get everything you want.

From my personal experience I know that everything I do more than 3-4 days   becomes a habit. So, if you use your will a few days to run the practices, they will become part of you in the coming days and you will make them naturally and with ease.

8TH STEP

Reporting the results and achievements of the work and efforts

You can make this step when 30 days past. Every day or every few days you can record in your diary everything that points or indicates the direction to achieve your goal.

When you have a specific purpose, the whole universe helps you to achieve it, so you should observe everything - the billboards that you pass by; the people you meet this month; books or magazines that you attract your attention. These are signals and signs that you're attracted to yourself with your thoughts and feelings. They will help you to find the easiest path and direction to materialize your goal.

If you follow the steps conscientiously you will be in synchronization with the higher consciousness. Everything you touch will be perfect and will happen in the best and the easiest way. There will be no tensions and difficulties. Just everything you want will happen like magic that comes for you.

The truth is that anything that is good for us and is in harmony with the higher mind   happens and comes to us. Try it and be amazed by the sophistication of the Universe. At the end of the month subscribe all the results and tell yourself that you are a perfect and unique person.

9TH STEP

We appreciate and reward ourselves for the success.

This step is my favourite one!

Now you can afford to reward yourself. Do not forget to thank yourself for the fact that you have taken a journey into yourself and you've overcome things that you bring with you so long. It is an incredible spiritual capital that you created for very little time when you could change even a small piece of you. You will be able to see and feel clearly how little we need sometimes to improve our lives!

Give yourself thanks and reward yourself!. Enjoy the achieved results. Make your desired holiday, alone or with your family and loved ones. Go to the cinema or to the theatre. Buy yourself a nice gift or flowers. Go to a special place for you in your dreams. Make a folly if it will bring you joy. Let all that you feel and makes you happy to happen to you!

CONCLUSIONS

Each of us has a unique personality!

The universe gives us limitless alternatives. Every time we have a choice that we do not always use, but we have it.

Allow yourself to feel that you are entitled to that choice, even if you think this is not so. Yes, it is true when you are in a difficult situation or have some diseases things seem hopeless. But the truth is that even then we have a choice. We can get angry, blame, curse fate or someone else, but we must try to see what we can learn in this very situation. However, this is a choice too, isn`t it?

Sometimes we can not change things so easily, but we can at least choose to seek and accept the gift of the fate even in difficulties and troubles. And in those moments of acceptance and humility a miracle always happens. We grow and improve our souls!!!

A great philosopher once said, "If we can overcome even a flaw in our life it is a great spiritual capital for our next rebirth." So I believe in that and I sincerely hope each of you will be able to win something in yourself and   allow the happiness and love to perform and accompany your life.

I wish you from deep in my heart to achieve any goal, any desire you have with ease! It could bring you all the joy, happiness and love in the world! Do not forget to thank each day that you are the most beautiful and perfect being. Love unconditionally and take care of yourself with all the love on which you are capable!

Yours

Amrit